DOGGY & ME

LUXDIOR.CO

Vol 2.

MASTER THE ART OF GOURMET PET CUISINE:

ELEVATE YOUR PUP'S DINING EXPERIENCE WITH EXPERT RECIPES

38 GOURMET
RECIPES FOR YOU & YOUR PUP

RAISE A PAW TO DOGGY HAPPY HOUR:

INDULGE YOUR PUP WITH LUX DIOR DOGGY BEER, BOW WOW BOURBON, DOG TEAQUILA...

THE ULTIMATE CANINE COCKTAILS!

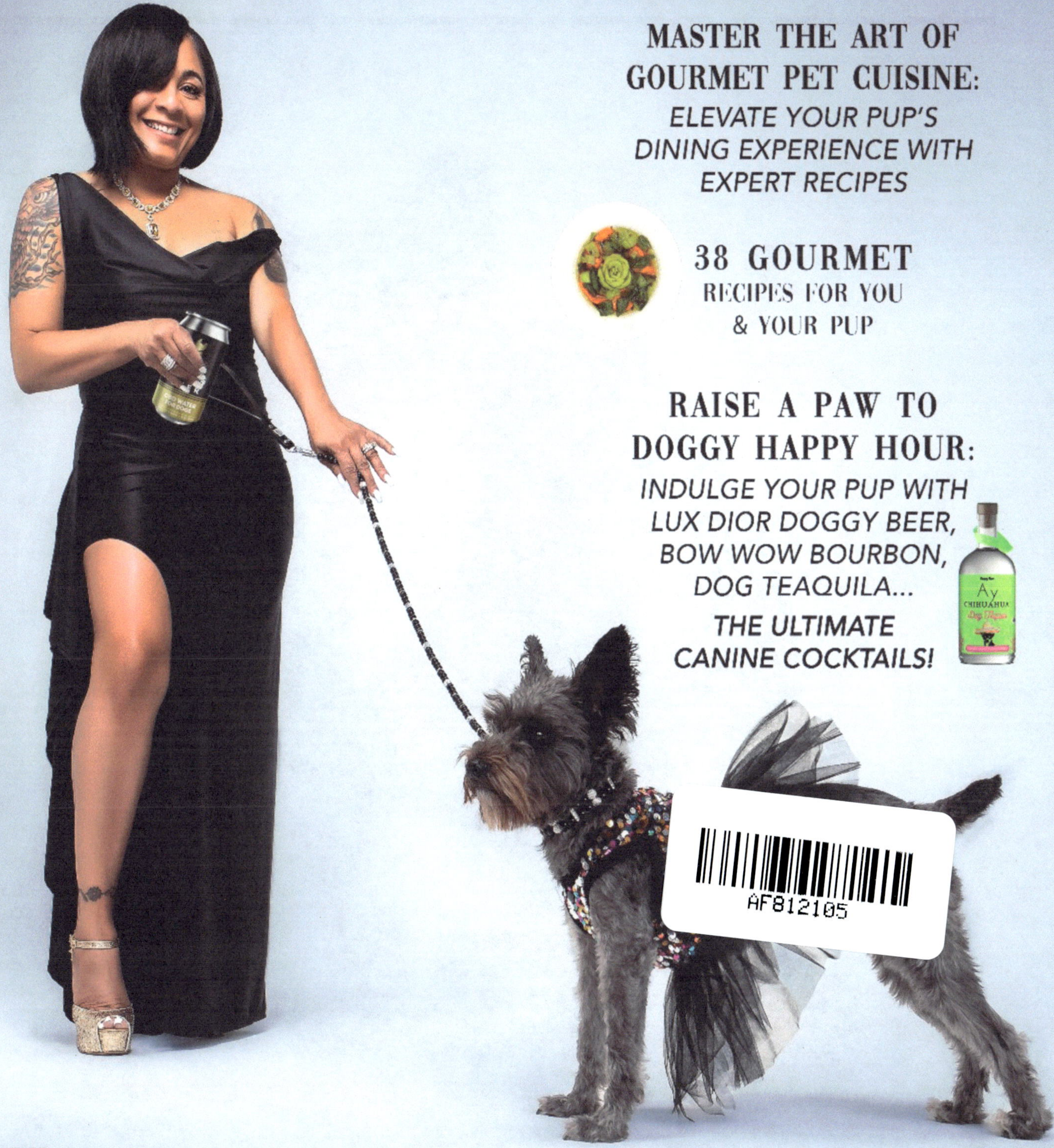

Follow us on
LUXDIOR.CO

LUXDIOR.CO
By Dee DeVaughn

TAILS & ALES

YOUR PUP'S FAVORITE TIME

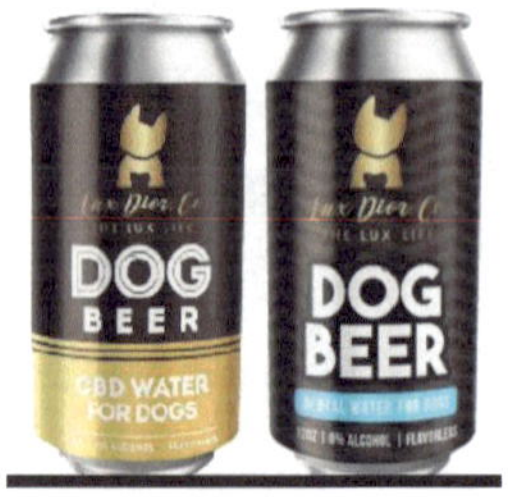

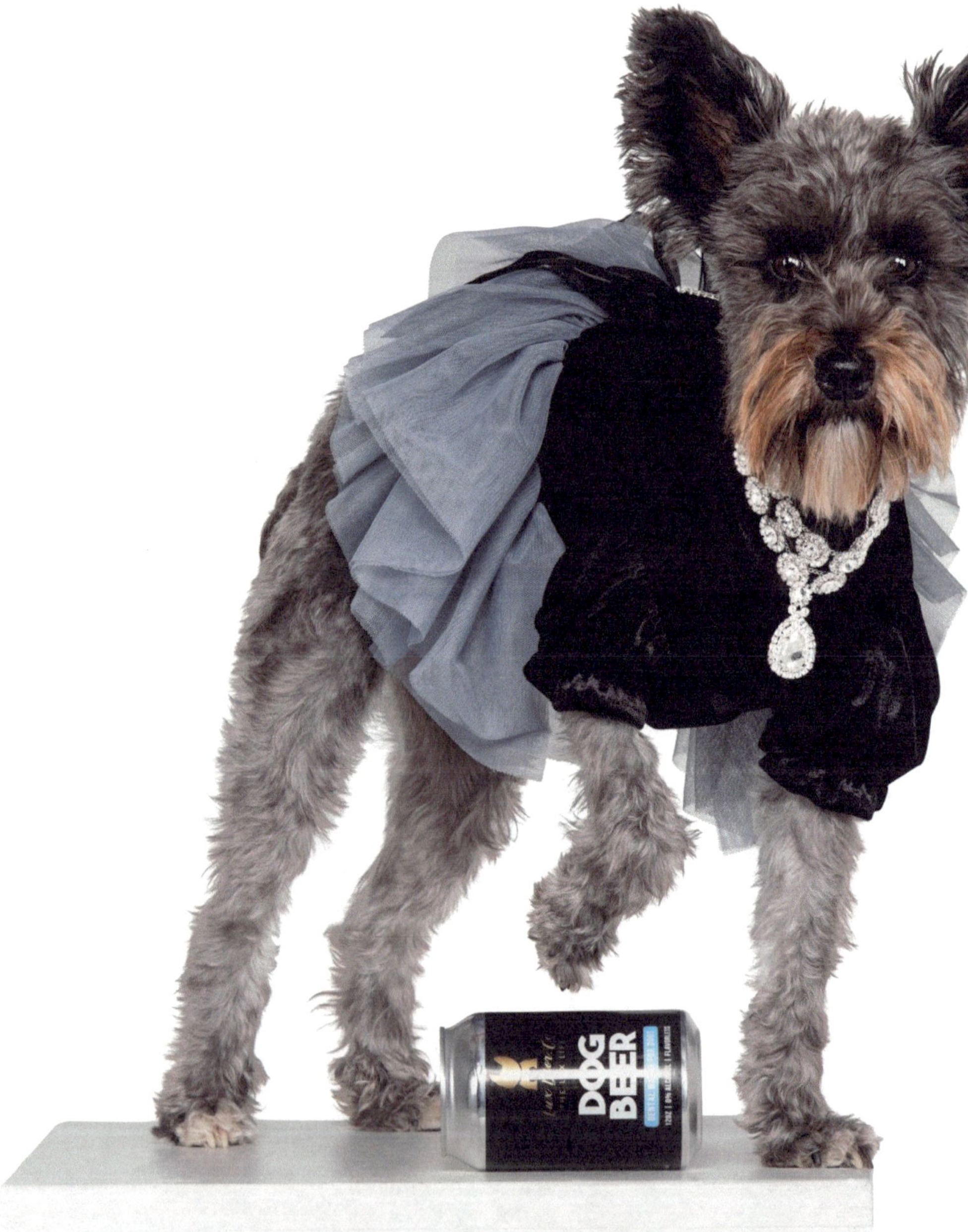

Lux Dior. Co
THE LUX LIFE

the

Cook Book

BK Royston Publishing
www.bkroystonpublishing.com

Cover Design and Interior Images: Miguel Hampton

Editor/Proofreader: JoAnn Hart and Jen Selinsky

ISBN-13: 978-1-963136-74-6

Printed in the United States of America

On behalf of Lux Dior Co *The Doggy & Me Cookbook*, a unique and exciting venture that aims to celebrate the joy of cooking for our furry companions.

The inspiration for this cookbook originated from my travels and dining experiences over the past year. I believe we all have experienced that one restaurant or meal that simply blew our minds and whether it was the flavors of a dish or the unforgettable service, it left a tasty memory for your pallet. I feel that our furry loved ones should have that same opportunity. When I prepare private dog dinners I set the mood for a four paws experience, linen on the table, flameless candlelight, charger plates, china, crystal, stemware anything and everything to set atmosphere. The dinners are 3-5 course meals paired with a suggested dog wine or specially crafted mocktail. Presenting delicious gourmet cuisine designed to pamper your pet like royalty. The Lux Dior brand is dedicated to elevating the lifestyle of any beloved furry friend.

The Doggy & Me Cookbook is a collection of recipes that brings together dog lovers and cooking enthusiasts alike. We inspire pet owners to create nutritious, delicious meals for their beloved canine companions that they too can enjoy. Our Lux Dior Co seasoning blends are human grade herbs and spices that support a healthy and delectable assortment of flavors, which makes preparing and enjoying these recipes so much easier.

Content

Content

Bok Choy & Carrot Soup

Lux Dior. Co Cookbook

Prep Time:	**Cook Time:**	**Serves:**
10 mins	20 mins, plus an extra 5 mins to cool	3 to 4

Things You Need:

2 cups
Bok choy (chopped)

1 cup
Carrots (diced)

4 cups
Vegetable broth

1 TBSP
Dog-On-Good

1 TBSP
Pup-elicious

Here's How:

1 In a stock pot, combine chopped bok choy, carrots,
1 tablespoon of Dog-On-Good,
1 tablespoon of Pup-elicious.

2 Pour in vegetable broth.

3 Bring to a boil, then lower heat and cook until veggies are tender.

4 Allow soup to cool and serve.

***Helpful Notes:**

Spring Rolls

Lux Dior. Co Cookbook

Prep Time:
10 mins

Cook Time:
10 mins, plus an extra 5 mins to cool

Serves:
3 to 4

Things You Need:

2 cups
Cabbage (shredded)

1/2 cup
Carrots (shredded)

1 TBSP
Cooking oil

Bowl of hot water

Rice paper

**Optional—add protein of choice*

1/2 TSP
Paw-rific

1 TBSP
Pup-elicious

Here's How:

1 In a bowl, combine cabbage, carrots, 1/2 teaspoon Paw-rific, 1 tablespoon of Pup-elicious and mix well.

2 In a sauté pan, add 1 tablespoon of coconut oil, or cooking oil of choice, heat at medium temperature.

3 Once pan is hot, add veggie mix and cook until tender.

4 Once tender, remove veggies from pan and allow to cool.

5 Dip rice paper in bowl of hot water until pliable.

6 Lay rice paper on a nonstick surface and add 2 tablespoons of veggie mix. Fold all corners of rice paper inward to create the spring roll.

7 In a skillet, add 3 tablespoons of coconut oil or cooking oil of choice. Ensure that the bottom of the skillet is coated. Fry each spring roll on all sides until golden brown.

8 Allow to cool and serve.

*

***Helpful Notes:**

Cucumber Sandwich

Lux Dior. Co Cookbook

Prep Time:	**Cook Time:**	**Serves:**
10 mins	2 mins	3 to 4

Things You Need:

1 Cucumber
(thinly sliced)

1 cup
Whipped
cream cheese

6 slices
Bread
(or egg white bread)

1 TSP
Paw-rific

1 TSP
Dill

**See egg white bread recipe*

Here's How:

1 Clean and slice cucumber longways (preferably thinly sliced).

2 In a bowl, mix whipped cream cheese, 1 teaspoon of Pup-elicious, and 1teaspoon dill. Mix well.

3 Lightly toast bread slices. Remove crust/edges (if using egg white bread slice in half to create two smooth sides).

4 Spread cream cheese on bread and then a layer of cucumber. Cut your sandwich into 2– 4 bites.

5 Ready to serve.

*Helpful Notes:

Vegetable Soup

Lux Dior. Co Cookbook

Prep Time:	**Cook Time:**	**Serves:**
10 mins	15 mins, plus an extra 5 mins to cool	3 to 4

Things You Need:

2 Zucchinis
(cut like spaghetti)

1 cup

Mushrooms (sliced)

1 cup

Peas and diced carrots

4 cups

Broth (bone, veggie, chicken or beef)

1 TBSP

Dog-On-Good

1 TBSP

Pup-elicious

**Optional – add protein of choice*

Here's How:

1 In a stock pot, add 4 cups of broth, 1 tablespoon of Dog-On-Good, 1 tablespoon pf Pup-elicious. Mix and bring to a boil.

2 Once broth starts to boil, add peas and carrots. Bring heat down to medium.

3 Continue to cook for about 5 minutes then add mushrooms and zucchini.

4 Once zucchini are fork tender, (This should take about 3 minutes.) Remove from heat.

5 Allow to cool and serve.

***Helpful Notes:**

Butternut Squash Puree

Lux Dior. Co Cookbook

Prep Time:	**Cook Time:**	**Serves:**
10 mins	15 mins	1to 2

Things You Need:

2 cups
Butternut squash
(cubed)

1/2 cup
Heavy cream
or goat milk

1 TBSP
Cinnamon

1 TSP
Paw-rific

Here's How:

1 On a cookie sheet, spread out squash. Sprinkle cinnamon and Paw-rific on top and bake at 400 for 15 minutes

2 In a blender, add roasted squash and heavy cream or goat milk.

3 Blend until smooth or (add more cream if needed).

4 Once blended smooth, pour into a bowl and enjoy.

5 You can also top with roasted pumpkin seeds.

***Helpful Notes:**

Zesty Potato Hash

Lux Dior. Co Cookbook

Prep Time:
10 mins

Cook Time:
20 mins, plus an extra 5 mins to cool

Serves:
2 to 3

Things You Need:

2 Large
Potatoes (cubed)

1/2 cup
Bell peppers (diced)
[green, red, yellow, or orange]

1 TBSP
Cooking oil

Optional—Add protein of choice

1 TSP
Paw-rific

1 TSP
Pup-elicious

1 TSP
Dog-On-Good

Here's How:

1 In a bowl, combine potatoes, bell peppers, 1 teaspoon of Paw-rific, 1 teaspoon of Pup-elicious, 1 teaspoon of Dog-On-Good and 1 tablespoon of cooking oil.
Mix well.

2 Spread potato mix evenly onto a nonstick cookie sheet.

3 Bake at 425 for 15– 20 minutes or (until potatoes are tender).

4 Once tender, remove from pan and allow to cool.

5 Enjoy!

***Helpful Notes:**

Sweet Potato Flats

Lux Dior. Co Cookbook

Prep Time:	**Cook Time:**	**Serves:**
10 mins	20 mins, plus an extra 5 mins to cool	4 to 5

Things You Need:

2 Large
Sweet potatoes
(Sliced longways 1 inch thick)

1 Apple (diced)

1/4 cup
Walnuts (chopped)

1 TBSP
Cinnamon

2 TBSP
Brown sugar

1 TBSP
Water

1 TSP
Paw-rific

Here's How:

1 Place sweet potatoes on non stick cookie sheet and bake at 425 for 15– 20 minutes

2 In a sauté pan, combine brown sugar, cinnamon, Paw-rific, and water. On low medium heat, stir until the consistency of syrup.

3 Add apple and nuts and continue to mix until diced apples and nuts are fully coated. Remove from heat.

4 Once sweet potatoes are tender, remove from pan and allow to cool.

5 Top sweet potatoes with apple blend drizzle with honey and serve.

*Helpful Notes:

Loaded Carrot Fries

Lux Dior. Co Cookbook

Prep Time:	**Cook Time:**	**Serves:**
10 mins	10 mins, plus an extra 5 mins to cool	3 to 4

Things You Need:

2 Large
Carrots
(Cut longways into 2 inch fries)

1 cup
Cooked Bacon Bits

1 cup
Shredded Cheese

1 TBSP
Cooking Oil

1 TSP
Dog-On-Good

Here's How:

1 On a non stick cookie sheet, place carrots. Drizzle carrots with olive oil and sprinkle on Dog-On-Good to taste. Bake at 425 for 15 minutes.

2 Once carrot are fork tender, move carrots to an oven safe serving dish.

3 Top carrots with bacon bits and cheese.

4 Bake for 5 more minutes to melt cheese.

5 Allow to cool and serve.

***Helpful Notes:**

Watermelon Salad

Lux Dior. Co Cookbook

Prep Time:	**Cook Time:**	**Serves:**
10 mins	0	3 to 4

Things You Need:

1 Watermelon
(cubed)

1/4 cup
Mint Leaves
(chopped)

1 cup
Feta cheese

Here's How:

1 Toss watermelon, mint leaves and feta cheese.

2 Plate and serve.

*Helpful Notes:

Barkognese Pasta

Lux Dior. Co cookbook

Prep Time:	**Cook Time:**	**Serves:**
10 mins	10 mins, plus an extra 5 mins to cool	3 to 4

Things You Need:

2 cups
Spinach

1 cup
Zucchini (cut)

1 cup
Bacon (cooked/crumbled)

1 cup
Egg noodles

1 TBSP
Cooking oil

1 TSP
Dog-On-Good

Here's How:

1 In a skillet, cook chopped bacon. In a pot, bring two cups of water to a boil then add egg noodles (cook until tender).

2 Remove the cooked bacon and add veggies to the same skillet (season and cook until spinach turns limp).

3 Once veggies are done, turn the heat to low and crumble bacon. Return bacon to the skillet.

4 Save 1/4 cup of pasta water and set to the side then drain the rest

5 Add noodles and pasta water to meat and veggies. Stir.

6 Allow to cool and serve.

*Helpful Notes:

Dior Shrimp Pasta

Lux Dior. Co cookbook

Prep Time:	**Cook Time:**	**Serves:**
10 mins	10 mins, plus an extra 5 mins to cool	3 to 4

Things You Need:

1/2 Pound
Shrimp

1 cup
Bok choy (chopped)

1 cup
Zucchini (diced)

1 cup
Egg Noodles

1 TBSP
Cooking oil

1 TSP
Dog-On-Good

Here's How:

1 In a non pan, add a drizzle of oil. Add zucchini, Bok choy, and seasoning.

2 In a pot, bring two cups of water to a boil. Add egg noodles.

3 Once veggies are tender, add shrimp and cook until shrimp is done.

4 Save 1/2 cup of pasta water, drain remaining water from noodles.

5 Add pasta water and noodles to a pan of meat and veggies.

6 Allow to cool and serve.

***Helpful Notes:**

Pupsagna

Lux Dior. Co cookbook

Prep Time:	Cook Time:	Serves:
10 mins	10 mins, plus an extra 5 mins to cool	3 to 4

Things You Need:

1 pound
Ground beef, Chicken or Lamb

1/2 cup
Beets (cooked)

1/2 cup
Pumpkin or Sweet Potato (mashed)

Lasagna pasta

2 oz
Goat cheese or cottage cheese

1 TSP
Dog-On-Good

1 TSP
Pup-elicious

Here's How:

1. In a skillet, brown and season meat. Drain and sit to the side.
2. Boil pasta until al dente.
3. Blend beets with pumpkin (or sweet potato) until smooth.
4. In an oven safe pan, layer pasta, meat, sauce, cheese and veggie. Repeat. (Two layers is recommended.) Optional: Top with shredded cheese.
5. Bake at 350 for 10 minutes.
6. Allow to cool and serve.

*Helpful Notes:

Pup Ramen

Lux Dior. Co cookbook

Prep Time:	**Cook Time:**	**Serves:**
5 mins	10 min,s plus an extra 5 mins to cool	1 to 2

Things You Need:

1 cup
Ramen or Greek egg noodles

2 cups
(Meat or Veggie broth)

1 cup
Chopped vegetables (celery, carrots, peas)

2 Boiled eggs

1 TSP
Dog-On-Good

1 TSP
Pup-elicious

**Optional—Add protein of choice*

Here's How:

1 In a pot, bring broth to a boil.

2 Add noodles to boiling water. Boil for about 3 minutes and then reduce heat.

3 Add veggies and pre cooked seasoned meat. Cook until veggies are tender.

4 Let stand and cool.

***Helpful Notes:**

Paw Puff

Lux Dior. Co cookbook

Prep Time:	**Cook Time:**	**Serves:**
10 mins	15 mins, plus an extra 5 mins to cool	4 to 6

Things You Need:

1 package
Puff Pastry

1 pound
Ground beef, pork, or chicken

1 cup
Cheese (shredded)

1 TBSP
Dog-On-Good

1 TBSP
Pup-elicious

Here's How:

1 Brown ground meat, season and drain of any oil.

2 Roll out puff pastry and cut into squares (the size of the square depends on how many you want to make).

3 Add pre cooked meat and cheese to the center of the puff pastry square and fold corners inward until completely closed.

4 Place on a nonstick cookie sheet (1+ inch apart). Bake at 400 for 15 minutes or until golden brown.

5 Allow to cool and serve.

***Helpful Notes:**

Loaded Nachos

Lux Dior. Co cookbook

Prep Time:	**Cook Time:**	**Serves:**
10 mins	6 mins, plus an extra 5 mins to cool	3 to 4

Things You Need:

2 Flour tortillas
(cut into 4 pieces)

1 cup
Bacon bits

1 cup
Cheese (shredded)

1 TSP
Dog-On-Good

Here's How:

1 Cut tortillas into four triangles. Cook at 350 for 3-4 minutes on a cookie sheet.

2 Top with a layer of cooked bacon bits and cheese.

3 Return to oven for 2 more minutes or until cheese melts.

4 Let stand and cool.

***Helpful Notes:**

Pizza

Lux Dior. Co cookbook

Prep Time:	Cook Time:	Serves:
10 mins	6 mins, plus an extra 5 mins to cool	3 to 4

Things You Need:

1 Flour tortilla
Spinach

2 TBSP
Pumpkin or Sweet potato puree

1/4 cup
Cheese (shredded)

1 oz
Turkey pepperoni

1 TBSP
Dog-On-Good

Here's How:

1. On a cookie sheet, add a tortilla, pumpkin or sweet potato puree, turkey pepperoni, and cheese.
2. Layer and cook in an oven at 350 for 6 minutes.
3. Cut into pizza slices.
4. Let stand and cool.

***Helpful Notes:**

Gumbo

Lux Dior. Co cookbook

Prep Time:	Cook Time:	Serves:
10 mins	10 mins, plus an extra 5 mins to cool	3 to 4

Things You Need:

1 cup of
Brown rice

2 cups of
Bone broth

1 stalk each of
Celery and Carrot (chopped)

1/2 cup of
Shrimp (cut and deveined)

1 cup of
Chicken (diced)

1 TSP
Beet powder

1 TBSP
Paw-rific

Here's How:

1 In a pot, bring broth and veggies to a boil.

2 Cook brown rice. Boil for about 10 minutes (al dente.)

3 In a skillet, sauté seasoned chicken and shrimp.

4 Combine broth and vegetable with beet powder.

5 Add protein and rice to the broth and vegetables. Stir.

6 Cool and serve.

***Helpful Notes:**

Salmon & Rice

Lux Dior. Co cookbook

Prep Time:	**Cook Time:**	**Serves:**
10 mins	15 mins, plus an extra 5 mins to cool	3 to 4

Things You Need:

8 oz. cut

Salmon

1 cup

Rice

2 cups of

Bone broth

1 cup of

Asparagus (cut)

1 TSP
Olive oil

1 TSP
Paw-rific,

1 TSP
Dog-On-Good

1 TSP
Pup-elicious

Here's How:

1 Drizzle seasoned salmon and asparagus with extra virgin olive oil.

2 Cook in oven or air fryer at 350 for 10-15 minutes.

3 Add rice and broth to pot and boil until rice is tender.

4 Add cooked salmon and asparagus to rice.

Let stand and cool.

***Helpful Notes:**

Surf & Turf

Lux Dior. Co cookbook

Prep Time:
10 mins

Cook Time:
10 mins, plus an extra 5 mins to cool

Serves:
3 to 4

Things You Need:

8 oz
Filet steak (or cut of choice)

4 large
Shrimp

2 medium
Potatoes

1 cup
Broccoli

1 TBSP
Olive oil

Seasonings
Paw-rific
Dog-On-Good
Pup-elicious

Here's How:

1 Drizzle olive oil on, and season, steak. Pan sear on both sides. Reduce heat to medium and continue to cook until medium well.

2 In separate pan, drizzle olive oil on shrimp, cook on medium heat for 5-7 minutes depending on size.

3 Boil potatoes for 10+ minutes or until fork tender.

4 Steam broccoli for 2-3 minutes.

5 Let stand and cool.

***Helpful Notes:**

Steak Fried Rice

Lux Dior. Co cookbook

Prep Time:
10 mins

Cook Time:
10 mins, plus an extra 5 mins to cool

Serves:
3 to 4

Things You Need:

4-6 oz
Filet steak (or steak of choice)

2 cups
Brown rice (cooked)

1 cup
Carrots (diced)

1 cup
Peas

1 TBSP
Olive oil

Seasonings
Paw-rific
Dog-On-Good
Pup-elicious

Here's How:

1 Drizzle olive oil on, and season, steak. Pan sear on both sides. Reduce heat to medium and continue to cook until medium well.

2 Drizzle olive oil in separate pan, medium heat add rice, carrots, peas, seasoning.

3 Cut steak into bite size pieces

4 Mix fried rice and steak in bowl.

5 Let stand and cool.

***Helpful Notes:**

Cheesy Meatball Pasta

Lux Dior. Co cookbook

Prep Time:	**Cook Time:**	**Serves:**
10 mins	10 mins, plus an extra 5 mins to cool	3 to 4

Things You Need:

1 pound
Ground beef

1 cup
Ditalini pasta

1 cup
Goat milk

1/2 cup
Shredded mozzarella cheese

1/4 cup
Cream cheese

Seasonings
Dog-On-Good
Pup-elicious

Here's How:

1 Season the ground beef and roll into small meatballs.

2 Place meatballs on a baking sheet and bake at 300 degrees for 15– 20 minutes.

3 Bring 2 cups of water to a boil, add pasta, and cook for 10 minutes or until al dente.

4 In a sauce pan, add a drizzle of olive oil, goat milk, cream cheese and shredded cheese.

5 Add pasta and meatballs to the cheese sauce.

6 Let stand and cool.

***Helpful Notes:**

Strawberry Cheesecake Ice Cream

Lux Dior. Co cookbook

Prep Time:	**Cook Time:**	**Serves:**
5 mins	0	3 to 4

Things You Need:

8 oz

Cottage cheese

1 oz

Whipped Cream cheese

1/3 cup

Strawberries (frozen)

Drizzle Honey or Maple syrup

1 TBSP
Water

Here's How:

1. In a blender, add cottage cheese, cream cheese, strawberries, water, and honey or maple syrup
2. Blend until smooth.
3. Add to a freezer safe container and freeze for 2-3 hours.
4. Bowl and serve cold.

***Helpful Notes:**

Watermelon Pawtini

Lux Dior. Co cookbook

Prep Time:	Cook Time:	Serves:
5 mins	0	1

Things You Need:

8 oz

Ay Chihuahua Dog

Tequila (puppy)

1/2 cup

Watermelon (cubed)

Here's How:

1 In a blender, add watermelon and puppy Tequila.

2 Blend until smooth.

3 Pour and serve.

4 Optional: add a small watermelon wedge.

***Helpful Notes:**

Carob Mousse

Lux Dior. Co cookbook

Prep Time:	**Cook Time:**	**Serves:**
5 mins	0	3 to 4

Things You Need:

8 oz
Cottage cheese

1 TBSP
Carob powder

Drizzle
Honey or Maple syrup

1 TSP
Water

Here's How:

1 In a blender, add cottage cheese, carob powder, water, honey or maple syrup

2 Blend until smooth.

3 Add to container and refrigerate for 1 hour

4 Bowl and serve.

***Helpful Notes:**

Chicken & Dressing

Lux Dior. Co cookbook

Prep Time:	Cook Time:	Serves:
25 mins	40 mins, plus an extra 5 mins to cool	3 to 4

Things You Need:

1 whole
Chicken (deboned)

2 cups
Corn meal

1 1/2 cups
Goat milk

2 Large
eggs

2 cups
Chicken broth

4 stalks
Celery (diced)

Seasonings
Dog-On-Good
Pup-elicious

Here's How:

1 In an oven safe pan, season and cook chicken at 350 for 30 minutes or until done.

2 Blend corn meal, egg, coconut oil, milk and add to a greased cast iron skillet. Cook in the oven at 400 degrees for 20-25 minutes.

3 In a skillet, cook celery with veggie broth. Season with Dog-On-Good and Pup-elicious seasonings.

4 Once corn bread is done, crumble in a large bowl, add celery mix and 1 egg. Mix well. (Add more veggie broth as needed for desired consistency.)

5 Move this mixture to an oven safe pan and cook for 15-20 minutes at 350 degrees.

6 Bring 2 cups of broth to a boil. Add 1-2 tbsp of flour and Thicken to consistency of gravy.

7 Dice cooked chicken and add gravy.

8 Allow to cool and serve.

***Helpful Notes:**

Pupkin pie

Lux Dior. Co cookbook

Prep Time:
10 mins

Cook Time:
15 mins, plus an extra 5 mins to cool

Serves:
3 to 4

Things You Need:

1 roll

Pie crust

1-16 oz Can

Pumpkin

1 Large

Egg

1 TSP

Honey

1/4 cup
Oat milk

Here's How:

1 In a greased mini muffin pan, add pie crust to each muffin cup cook for 6 minutes at 350 degrees.

2 Blend pumpkin, egg, honey, cinnamon, and oat milk.

3 Add pumpkin mix to each muffin cup.

4 Bake at 350 degrees for 15 minutes.

5 Allow to cool and serve.

***Helpful Notes:**

Turkey Potpie

Lux Dior. Co cookbook

Prep Time:	**Cook Time:**	**Serves:**
5 mins	60 mins, plus an extra 5 mins to cool	3 to 4

Things You Need:

1 pound
Turkey (Cubed)

1 cup
Carrots, peas
Potatoes (diced)

2 rolls
Pie crust

1-2 cups
Turkey broth

Here's How:

1 Add turkey to oven safe pan and cook at 350 for 30-40 minutes.

2 In a pot on medium, add mixed veggies and heat.

3 In a deep dish, add pie crust and bake for 15 minutes at 350 degrees.

4 In sauce pan, bring turkey broth to a boil and add 1-2 tbsp of flour to thicken for gravy.

5 In cooked pie shell, add turkey, veggies and gravy. Top with a sheet of pie crust.

6 Place back into oven for 20 minutes.

6 Allow to cool and serve.

***Helpful Notes:**

Pawberry Punch

Lux Dior. Co cookbook

Prep Time:	Cook Time:	Serves:
5 mins	0	1

Things You Need:

4 oz

Bow Wow Bourbon (puppy)

4 oz

Ay Chihuahua Dog

Tequila (puppy)

1 cup

Mixed fruit

Here's How:

1 In a blender, add mixed fruit, bourbon and tequila.

2 Blend until smooth.

3 Pour and serve.

*Helpful Notes:

Banana Forester

Lux Dior. Co cookbook

Prep Time:	**Cook Time:**	**Serves:**
5 mins	0	1

Things You Need:

8 oz

Bow Wow Bourbon (puppy)

1/4 cup

Banana

Drizzle

Honey or Maple syrup

Here's How:

1 In a blender, add Bourbon, bananas, honey or maple syrup.

2 Blend until smooth.

3 Pour and serve.

*Helpful Notes:

Paw Apple Mule

Lux Dior. Co cookbook

Prep Time:	**Cook Time:**	**Serves:**
5 mins	0	1

Things You Need:

8 oz
Ay Chihuahua Dog
Tequila (puppy)

1/2 cup
Apple sauce

Dash
Cinnamon

Here's How:

1 In a blender, add Tequila, apple sauce, cinnamon.

2 Blend until smooth.

3 Pour and serve.

***Helpful Notes:**

Peach Smash

Lux Dior. Co cookbook

Prep Time:	**Cook Time:**	**Serves:**
5 mins	0	1

Things You Need:

8 oz

Bow Wow Bourbon (puppy)

1/4 cup

Peaches (frozen)

Drizzle

Honey or Maple syrup

Here's How:

1 In a blender, add bourbon, peaches, maple syrup.

2 Blend until smooth.

3 Pour and serve.

***Helpful Notes:**

Tequila Tail Wag

Lux Dior. Co cookbook

Prep Time:	**Cook Time:**	**Serves:**
5 mins	0	1

Things You Need:

8 oz

Ay Chihuahua Dog

Tequila (puppy)

1/4 cup

Pineapple (frozen

1/4 cup

Red berries (frozen

Here's How:

1 In a blender, add tequila, pineapple and red berries.

2 Blend until smooth.

3 Pour and serve.

***Helpful Notes:**

Tail Spin

Lux Dior. Co cookbook

Prep Time:	**Cook Time:**	**Serves:**
5 mins	0	1

Things You Need:

8 oz.
Lux Dior Dog Beer
CBD water (puppy)

1/4 cup
Strawberries (frozen)

1/4 cup
Bananas (frozen)

Here's How:

1 In a blender, add CBD beer, strawberries and bananas.

2 Blend until smooth.

3 Pour into cup or bowl and serve.

*Helpful Notes:

Paw Chatta

Lux Dior. Co cookbook

Prep Time:	Cook Time:	Serves:
5 mins	0	1

Things You Need:

8 oz.
Ay Chihuahua Dog
Tequila (puppy)

1 TBSP
Honey

1 TBSP
Coconut cream

Dash
Cinnamon

Here's How:

1. In a blender, add tequila, coconut cream, honey and cinnamon.
2. Blend until smooth.
3. Pour into cup/bowl and serve.

*Helpful Notes:

Fresh Breath Mojito

Lux Dior. Co cookbook

Prep Time:	**Cook Time:**	**Serves:**
5 mins	0	1

Things You Need:

8 oz

Lux Dior Dog Beer

Dental water (puppy)

1/4 cup

Cucumber

4 fresh

Mint leaves

Here's How:

1 In a blender, add beer, cucumber and mint leaves.

2 Blend until smooth.

3 Pour into cup/bowl and serve.

***Helpful Notes:**

LIC (Long Island Canine)

Lux Dior. Co cookbook

Prep Time:	**Cook Time:**	**Serves:**
5 mins	0	1

Things You Need:

8 oz.

Bow Wow Bourbon (puppy)

2 oz.

Bone broth

Here's How:

1 In a blender, add puppy bourbon and bone broth.

2 Blend until smooth.

3 Pour into cup/bowl and serve.

***Helpful Notes:**

Apple Tart

Lux Dior. Co cookbook

Prep Time:	Cook Time:	Serves:
5 mins	0	1

Things You Need:

1 Pastry pie shell

1 Apple (peeled and sliced)

Honey (drizzle)

1 tsp Cinnamon

Here's How:

1 In a bowl, mix apple, honey and cinnamon

2 Spoon mixture into pie shell.

3 Serve.

***Helpful Notes:**

Egg White Bread

Lux Dior. Co cookbook

Prep Time:	**Cook Time:**	**Serves:**
10mins	30 mins	2

Things You Need:

6 Large
Eggs

Drizzle
Maple syrup/honey

Here's How:

1 In a glass bowl, separate yokes from egg whites.

2 Blend until egg whites look like clouds.

3 Drizzle in maple syrup/ honey and continue to blend.

4 Once egg foam is of a thick consistency, place mounds onto a parchment lined baking sheet.

5 Allow space between each mound and bake at 350 degrees for 30 mins.

6 Allow to cool and serve.

***Helpful Notes:**

Benefits of Our Spices:

Pup-elicious

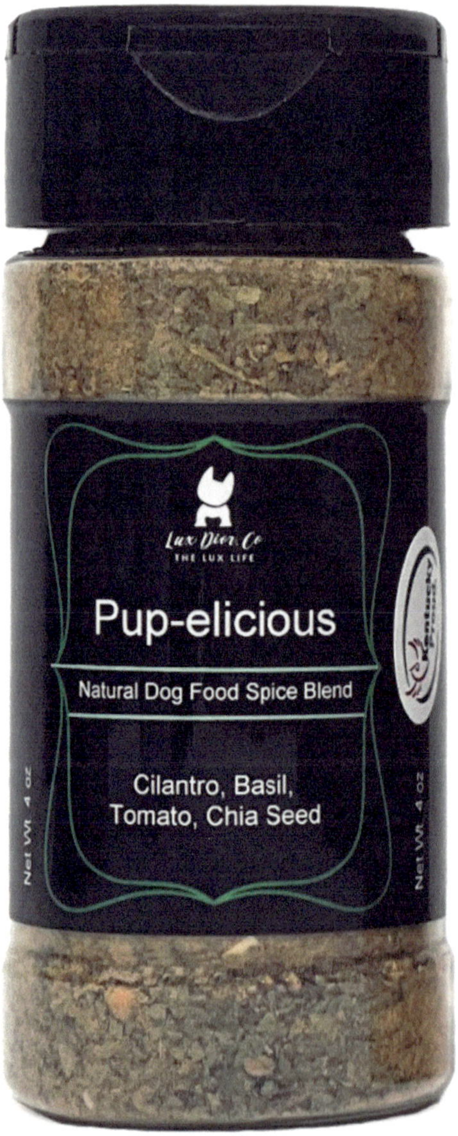

Cell Development

Digestive System

Immune System

Tissue Growth

Skin

Fur

Bone

Benefits of Our Spices:

Paw-rific

Anti-Inflammatory

Digestive Health

Immune System

Joints

Skin

Coat

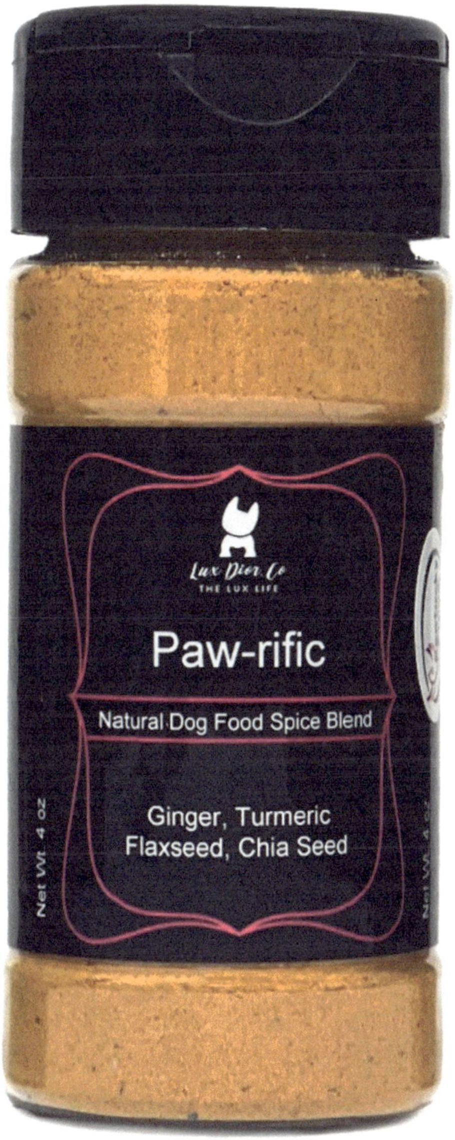

Benefits Of Our Spices:

Dog-On-Good

Heart Health

Immune System

Digestive System

Vision

Bone

Mood

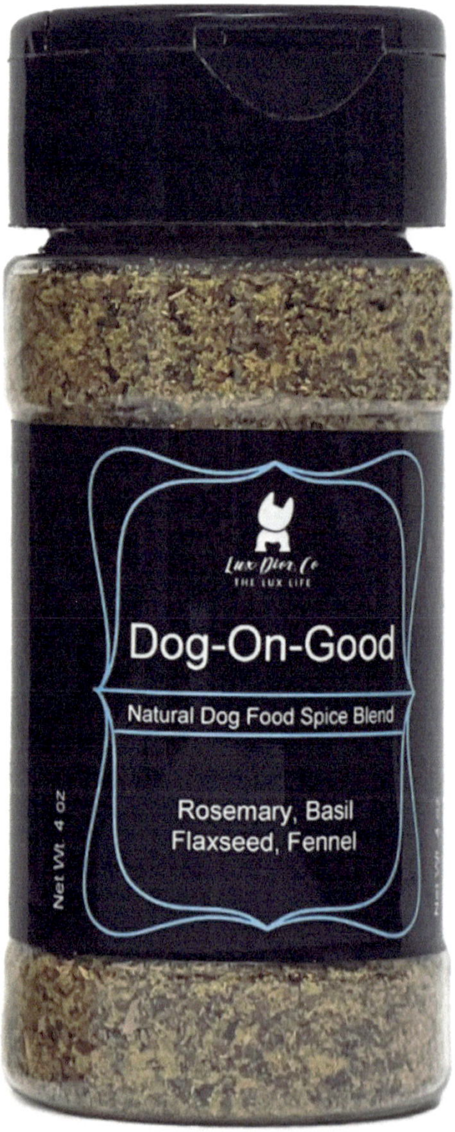

Lux and I wanted to take a moment to express our heartfelt gratitude for your incredible support of our cookbook and brand. Your enthusiasm and encouragement means the world to us.

Thank you for being a part of our journey and for believing in what we do. We're excited to continue bringing you delicious recipes and inspiration.

Warmest regards,
Dee DeVaughn & Lux Dior

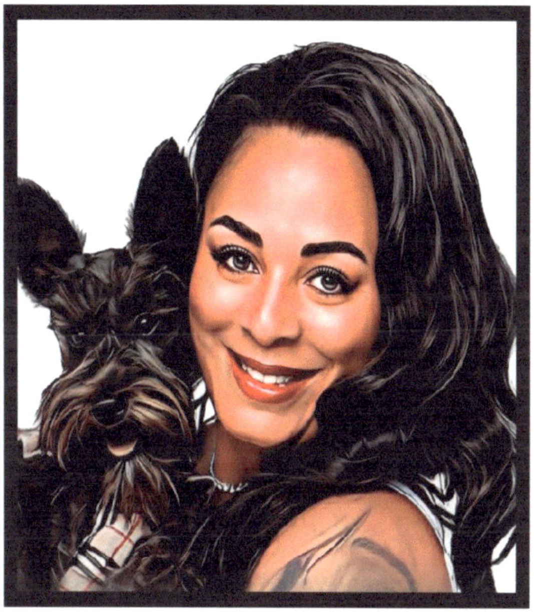

Connect with us on social media:
Instagram: @Luxdior.co
Facebook: LuxDior.co
Youtube.com/@LuxDior
TikTok: @Luxdior.co
Website: LuxDiorco.com

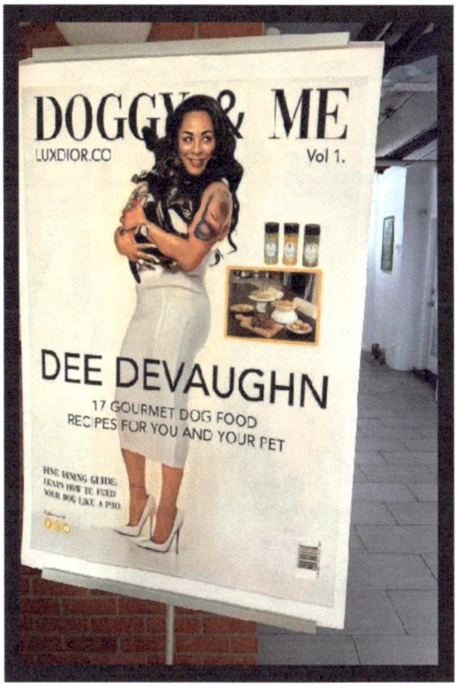

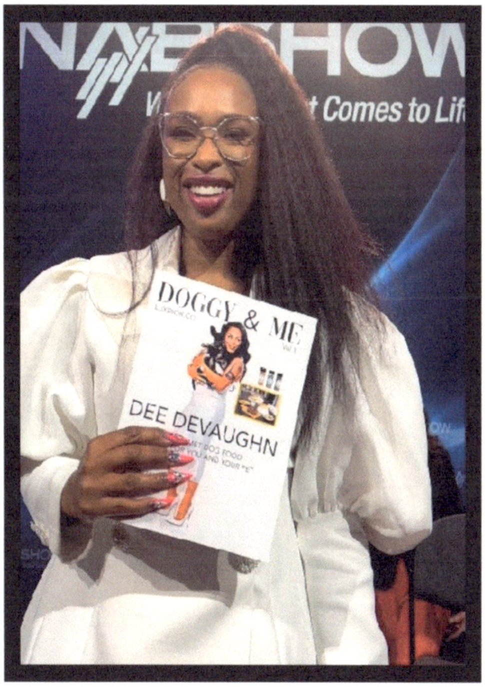

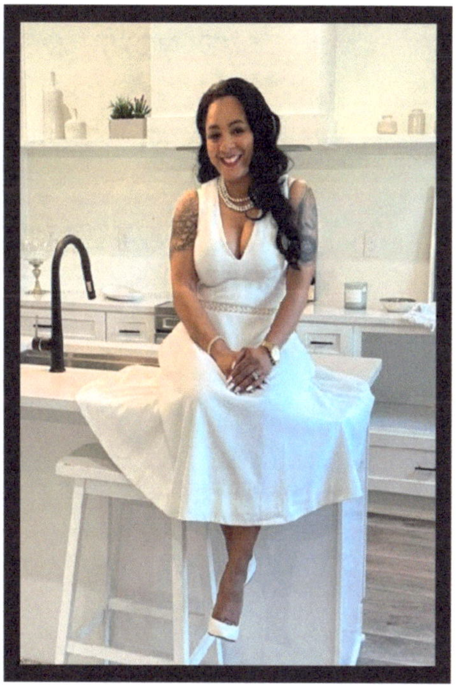

Welcome to Lux Dior. Co Dog Café!

Where every tail wags with joy!

At Lux Dior. Co, we specialize in "The Lux Life" with the companionship of furry friends. Enjoy our cozy atmosphere, sip on freshly brewed coffee, and indulge in private dog-friendly dinners, treats and mocktails while your pup socializes with fellow canines. Whether you're looking for a place to unwind or want to make new friends both human and canine!

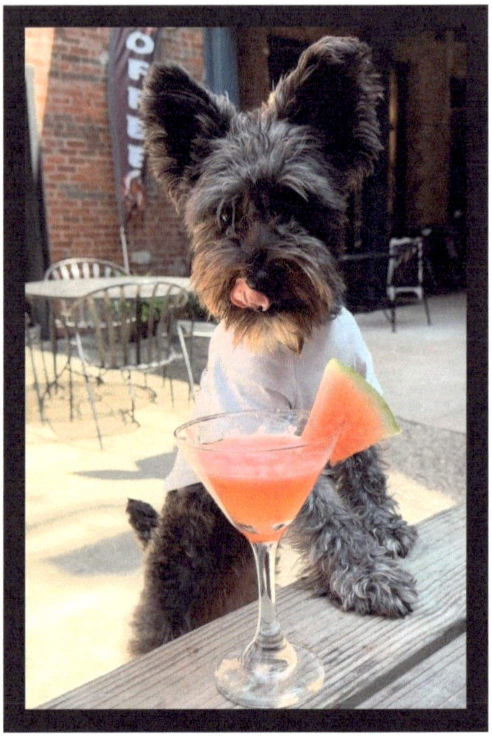

We've got you covered.

Bring your dog, relax and let the good times roll!

Visit us today at 1860 Mellwood Ave., Suite 115, Louisville Kentucky 40206 and discover your new favorite hangout spot. Don't forget to share your moments with us on social media using @LuxDior.Co.

Come in today—your new friends are waiting!

Lux Dior. Co

THE LUX LIFE

Made in the USA
Monee, IL
05 November 2026

67811008R00050